Producing Positivity

31 Days to a New Positive You

By

Joel T. Whiteside MSPC, LAC

Contents

You are loved and worthy of positive things in your life.

You have the power inside of you to produce it.

Let's go find it together.

Written in Honor Of

This book is written in memory of all those who have given up on life as a result of overwhelming negative circumstances and the inability to manifest positivity in the dark times. Also, to my mother, Ellie Whiteside, aka "Mama El", who always spoke positivity into my life. She passed away too early, but her spirit continues to inspire me in all areas of my life. "Love and Lollipops" to you forever.

Special thanks to Jolene, my wife, and best friend. Your unconditional love and support are second to none. You are my rock. Also, to my father Jerry, sister Jayme, ALL my special aunties who have stepped up to become mother figures, my extended family, and my TRIBE. Every one of you have played a special role in my life and have believed in me on the days I have trouble believing in myself. Thanks to my daughters Abbie and Kelsee. You both inspire me to be better and to have a positive impact in the world you will grow up in and raise your kids in. Lastly, I want to give all the glory to God for pulling me out of the darkness so I could shine light and serve others.

Introduction

This book is intended to help you move away from negativity and produce positivity in your life. It was inspired by the realization of how much more enjoyable life is when we live in a positive mindset. I don't believe I am alone when I say, "The world can be a very negative place, and sometimes our perspective lacks positivity". We inherently have a negative brain bias and will default to a negative thought pattern. We spend a tremendous amount of our lives viewing things through a lens of the glass is half empty, not half full. We must put forth effort to change our perception and begin seeing things through a positive set of lenses. All you will need to embark on this journey is 15 minutes of your time daily, something to write with, a few packs of sticky notes, and a willing heart. If you are reading this in ebook form, you will need a notebook and sticky notes. When you are tasked with writing you will use your notebook. Label each day with the topic and date. I am grateful you are on the path to positivity with us and excited about what the future holds for you. Let's do it and do it together.

The information and tasks presented in this book are designed in their most simplistic and usable form. The intent is for all age groups and people with different educational backgrounds to benefit. You won't be WOWED with a bunch of factual information, but you will be impacted by a WAVE of positive-provoking thoughts, insights, experiences, and suggestions. The hope is as you set your intentions each day in a positive direction, and incorporate simple practices, you will produce positivity in your life and those around you. Let's Go!

"Our mind tends to wander to dark and negative places as a result of our past experiences. When we validate or believe this negative pattern of thought, our behaviors will follow down a negative path. What we believe has power, and subsequently what we believe has power over us. Lining our spirit up with a more positive belief system, and a positive pattern of thought, has the potential to set us on a beautiful path of positivity we only dreamed of."

- Joel T. Whiteside

Intentions - Day 1

Intentions – Day 1

Intentions are goals we established, living in the same space as passion and desire. Setting goals can be a waste of energy if we don't believe in our hearts they will manifest into existence. At our core, we all want good things to happen in our lives, but simultaneously we live in doubt they will come to fruition. This negative mindset and conflicted spirit will continue to produce negative outcomes. Speaking goals into existence with the intention of completing them, and believing we will, inspires us to do our part and allow the universe or our Higher Power to support the process. Setting intentions every day to experience love, connection, happiness, gratitude, serenity, peace, and countless other positive principles will take us to a new level of existence. Wayne Dyer states, "The power of intention is the power to manifest, to create, to live a life of unlimited abundance, and to attract into your life the right people at the right moments."

Here are a few statements to set our intentions and incorporate into our morning routine. Find a quiet place free of distractions and repeat these statements out loud with conviction.

- Today I intend to be actively grateful for the things I have in my life.
- Today I intend to create positive social connections that are authentic and enrich my spirit.

- Today I intend to do good deeds and poor positivity into the world around me.
- Today I intend to lift myself up and speak life into my heart and mind.

Intentions aren't something we set on January 1st and ride the wave of positivity for the next 364 days. We must set intentions daily and follow through with them to create the life we truly deserve to experience. Above, we were provided with a list of intentions for today. Below we will develop a list of intentions for ourselves. You are encouraged to use this list you create for the following 7 days and slowly add and change it as the days go on.

1.) _____

2.) _____

3.) _____

With a daily practice of intention setting, we will begin to feel inspired to be the person we have always wanted to be. The masks we have created to protect ourselves will come off, and opportunities, experiences, relationships, gifts, restoration, and happiness will become mainstays in our day-to-day affairs. If you have a hard time believing this can come true, start by setting your intention to believe that WE believe.

"We know there is intention and purpose in the universe, because there is intention and purpose in us."

- George Bernard Shaw.

Progress Not Perfection-Day 2

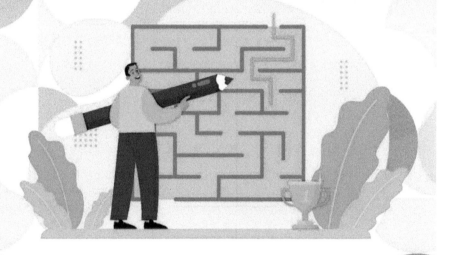

Progress Not Perfection – Day 2

Moving towards a more positive lifestyle isn't about perfection. Our goal is progress. We put unrealistic expectations on ourselves to achieve some monumental level of change without any issues along the way. Reality check…life isn't easy, nor is change. We have been stuck in a rut of negative thinking, feelings, and behaviors for an extended amount of time. The information we have received over the years results in negative core beliefs and barriers to our development. If we were told, "failure isn't an option," "second place is the first loser," or "you always mess things up," we tend to be extremely critical of ourselves and look at anything less than perfect as a bad thing. Winston Churchill stated, "Perfection is the enemy of progress." Moving away from our irrational beliefs of perfection, opens the door for us to progress in the direction our hearts desire.

The route to a positive life is to address things head-on and move right through the discomfort. In this process, we will fall short, bang our heads against the wall, backslide at times, and may create a little wreckage. This is part of the process, and learning is growing. There will be days when we are riding the positivity wave and others when we crash on the beach. Riding the wave provides us with the opportunity to live in gratitude. Crashing on the beach is an opportunity to regroup, reassess, and reestablish our plan.

Both circumstances produce positive progress and are equally beneficial.

Today we will set out with the intention to embrace challenges, failures, and times of adversity as opportunities to progress in a positive direction. We will begin to set realistic expectations of ourselves and give ourselves the same grace we give others. Frank Zappa stated, "Without deviation from the norm, progress is not possible." Below is a series of statements to begin to change the dialogue in our brains. Negative self-talk is the enemy of positive progress. We will read these out loud three different times throughout the day. In the future, when we find ourselves having unrealistic expectations or negative thinking, we will come back to these statements as a tool to shift to a more positive thought pattern. We can use the notes section in the book to develop our own statements if we would like.

1.) I will embrace life as it comes and not expect myself to be perfect.

2.) I am a fallible human being who is doing my best to progress forward in life.

3.) I will treat myself with the same grace, respect, and forgiveness I do with others.

4.) I will fall short regularly. And when I do, I will embrace the opportunity to be better.

5.) I am powerful, courageous, and willing to overcome adversity and challenges.

Some days we will take five steps forward and two back. Some days we will take one step forward and two steps back. There will be days when we don't even get off the start line. Regardless of how our day unfolds, there are opportunities to progress. At the end of the day, we will use the space below to identify areas we have made progress in. It is imperative we don't minimize the magnitude of any progress we make. Every step is important, even if we take three backwards. The path to positivity requires us to lift ourselves up and validate all our wins.

1.) _____

2.) _____

3.) _____

4.) _____

5.) _____

I believe in you and the potential for continued progress on this path to positivity. You aren't perfect, but you are an amazing person worthy of a positive life. Let's go out and get it.

"Progress means getting nearer to the place you want to be." – C.S. Lewis

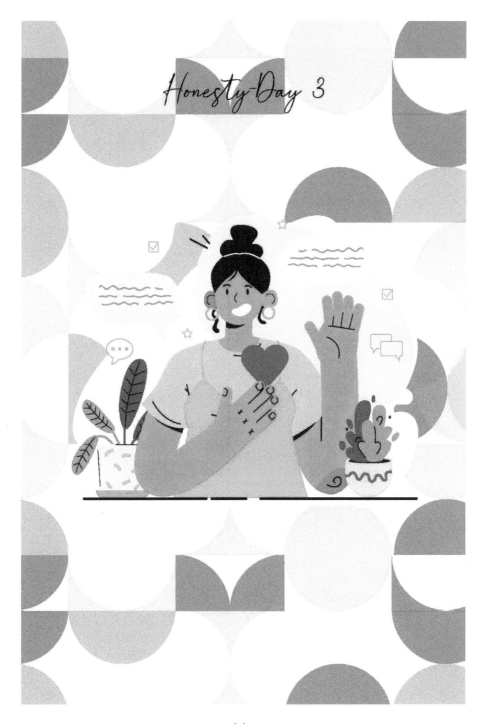

Honesty Day 3

Honesty – Day 3

Not all of us are raised to truly understand honesty, or have the ability to practice it. We are conditioned to be dishonest from a young age by our parents and family members. We hear things like, "don't show your feelings…it's a sign of weakness", or "don't tell your mom we just spent money on those toys". On the playground, we hear, "snitches get stitches" or "don't tell Sally I was holding hands with Susie". We are naturally born to be honest individuals, but we learn dishonesty through nurturing and our environment. Movies, social media, TV Shows, and society provide us with countless examples of the benefits of being dishonest. How could we not be influenced in some capacity by all this information we are receiving? The truth is we can't, and if we don't have positive influences in our lives, we are destined to develop a level of dishonesty.

There are several different types of dishonesty. All of these are not okay, by the way! We lie by omission and leave out a little bit of information in a story to avoid accepting responsibility. Yiddish Proverb states, "A half truth is a whole lie." In other cases, we just flat out lie to save our face, or image to look cool. I call this the "Ego Lie". There is also self-betrayal or being dishonest with ourselves. This may be the most impactful of all lies.

Today we set out with the intention of practicing honesty with others and ourselves. You may ask, how is this going to produce positivity in my life? Do you want me to tell on myself? Yes, that is what I am suggesting, but if you choose to continue to be dishonest, that is your prerogative. Each lie we have told or are currently holding onto is like a rock in our bag of life. The longer we hold onto these lies increases the weight of our bag. Let's lessen the load today and take some weight out. Starting small is key, and please don't admit to anything that will cause harm to you or others this early in the process.

We will start by establishing two areas we have been dishonest with ourselves about and write them down in the space below.

1.) _____

2.)_____

Just by writing these down and putting them into the universe, you have been honest with yourself. Your bag just got lighter.

Now we will identify two things we have been dishonest with others about and write them down in the space below.

1.) _____

2.) _____

Writing these down was the second step to lessening the load of rocks you are carrying. Now it is time to be courageous and go out and get honest! Opportunities to be honest will present themselves in your life and your relationships because you have set your intentions to be honest. Awareness is the key to change…today we move towards honesty. Let's do this….I believe in you.

"Honesty is more than not lying. It is truth telling, truth speaking, truth living, and truth loving." - James E. Faust

Surrender-Day 4

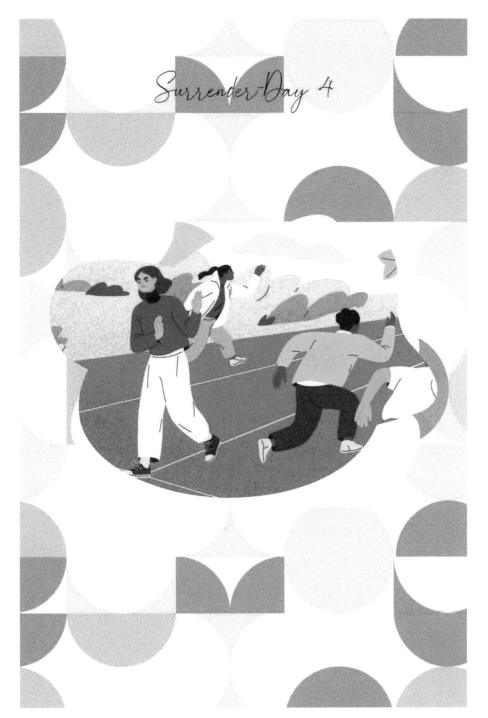

Surrender – Day 4

Surrender provides us with the opportunity to reach a level of peace, serenity, and positivity we have only dreamed of in the past. Certain beliefs and values we grew up with no longer serve us. In many cases, we have developed fixed ideas of how things need to be, should be, must be, and will always be because it provides safety for us. Anything outside of what we determine to be "okay" creates discomfort and a negative response we are unwilling to deal with. We attempt to fix, manage, and control everything in our lives to feel like we "have it going on." When in all reality, we are lost, confused, fearful, and overwhelmed. Some of us are willing to go to any lengths to hold on to things, and surrender isn't an option. Asking for help, giving up the fight, and being open to new ideas is seen as a sign of weakness. Sissy Gavrilaki said, "Sometimes, it's not the times you decide to fight, but the times you decide to surrender, that makes all the difference." Rigidity robs us of serenity, and without serenity, we lack the opportunity for positivity. We must be willing to surrender.

Throwing in the towel or raising the white flag are historically looked at as losing the battle. When the battle is one that will never end, surrendering is the only way to win. Practicing humility, surrendering, and asking for help are some of the most courageous things we will ever do. We don't have to be right all the time in order to come out on top. It is okay not to know or understand things. The admittance of this is a sign of strength, not weakness. Eckhart Tolle said, "Sometimes surrender means giving up trying to understand and becoming comfortable with not knowing." When we open ourselves up to different perspectives, and allow others to be a part of our journey, the opportunity for a positive life will multiply exponentially.

Today we will set our intentions to invite surrender into our lives, and become willing to let go of control. The trajectory of our life can change drastically if we surrender to a new way of living. Identification is a key to change, and today we are only beginning the process. We will start this by identifying 3-5 different things, ideas, people, fears, beliefs, or resentments we are holding onto and write them down in the space provided.

1.) _____

2.) _____

3.) _____

4.) _____

5.) _____

The identification of these things will ultimately present us with opportunities in the future to surrender, ask for help, and begin to let go. We need to take advantage of these times. We must become vulnerable and invite people into our process. Our lives become richer and more enjoyable when we are surrounded with the support and love of others. I am excited to see the maturation of your surrender process over the course of this 31 day adventure. Lets make it happen!

"Change is the essence of life; be willing to surrender what you are for what you could become." - Reinhold Niebuhr

Vulnerability-Day 5

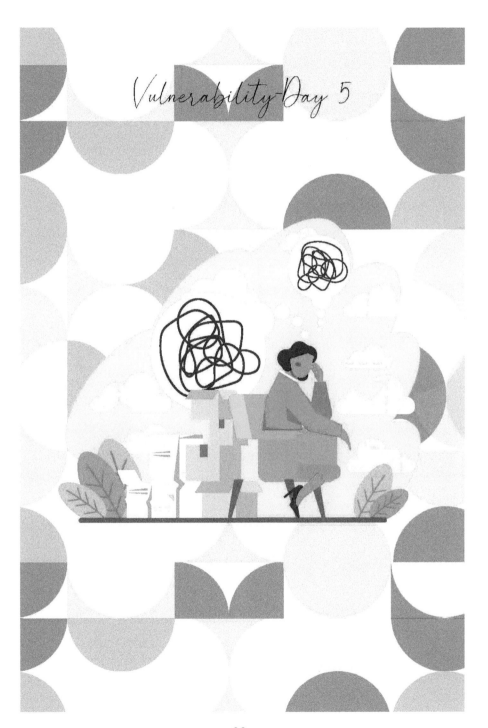

Vulnerability – Day 5

The word vulnerability itself may make you cringe and create a negative pattern of thoughts. Many of us have developed core beliefs that we can't trust people or share our authentic selves because we will get hurt. These feelings are valid, and we maintain a sense of safety by keeping the walls up around us. These walls protect us and keep others from getting to know us and potentially hurting us. Consequently, they also keep us locked in a self-made prison and rob us of our opportunity to benefit from social connection. We need each other, and we depend on social connections to truly feel a sense of love and belonging. Brene Brown states, "I define vulnerability as uncertainty, risk, and emotional exposure. To be human is to be in vulnerability." I am assuming if you are reading this....you are a human. Now that we have established that, let's be courageous humans today and share our true selves with other humans.

"Be yourself, everyone else is already taken."

- Oscar Wilde

Today's intentional task is simple. First, we must lower our walls, and become willing to share our true selves with others. I assume there are things you have been holding onto or are renting space in your heart because being vulnerable is risky. This may be pain around current circumstances you are trying to carry yourself. It could be a crush you have on someone, but are scared to share it with them out of fear of rejection. Maybe it's the frustration you have with your partner around their lack of attention to you, and you don't want to rock the boat. This may be your need to ask for help with a project at work, but your ego is in the way. You may be struggling with sadness, anxious feelings, or feeling empty inside, but don't want to reach out due to fear of judgment. Regardless of the circumstance, today is the day we let the walls down and allow others a glimpse of our true self.

On the lines below, briefly establish two situations you will practice vulnerability in today, or walls you will let down. Lets be courageous!

1.) _____

2.) _____

We no longer need to hide behind imaginary walls. Sheltering ourselves from the world around us out of fear of being hurt, will also shelter ourselves from experiencing love. Today we open up the door to the world by opening ourselves up to the idea of being vulnerable, and putting it into practice. This is the beginning of a lifelong process of deconstructing the walls we have built. As time progresses, we will find it easier to open up, be authentic, and be vulnerable. It all starts with today….Lets go!

"Freedom is not worth having if it does not include the freedom to make mistakes."

- Mahatma Gandhi

Dreams Day 6

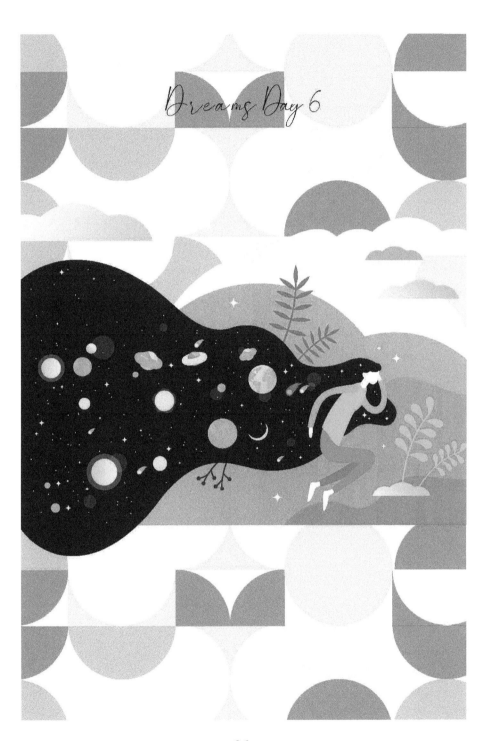

Dreams – Day 6

Dreams will never become a reality if we don't follow them up with action. From a young age, we all dreamed of being something. Nurses, Lawyers, Doctors, Mechanics, Police Officers, Firefighters, Ironworkers, Business Owners, etc. In many cases, we follow in our parents' or role models' footsteps because certain careers are generational, or we are conditioned to believe this is what we do. In this process, we lose connection with what we really want in life and find ourselves in a box we don't want to be in. In other instances, we put limiting beliefs on ourselves as a result of our socioeconomic class, ethnicity, gender, criminal history, family history, or level of education. We say things like, "I could never do that, people like me never succeed." We all have so much potential, but as a result of past experiences we live in fear of failure, fear of a challenge, and fear of the work it will take to achieve our dreams. Safe is safe, but it sets us up for being mediocre and lacking contentment. Eric Thomas said, "You cannot afford to live in the potential phase for the rest of your life; at some point you have to unleash the potential and make your move." Today is the day we will begin the process of making our move.

We will set our intentions today to establish dreams far beyond what we are currently doing and then begin to believe we can achieve them. This isn't an assignment to identify things we can easily accomplish. That is safe, and remember, safe creates mediocre. This is a list to identify the things deep in our hearts we want to do but never thought possible. This is a list of things people around us say we can't do. These are things stereotypically people like us don't do. We aren't put on this earth to live in a box that society, our parental figures, or peers put us in. We are given the opportunity to be who we want to be and impact the world on a larger scale than we ever thought possible.

When writing down your list below, "I am going to…." is attached to each line. This is your intentional commitment to yourself, the world, and your Higher Power of what you are going to do…and no longer just dream about.

1.) I am going to

_____

2.) I am going to

_____

3.) I am going to

_____

4.) I am going to

_____

5.) I am going to

_____

We have now intentionally established what our dreams are, and made the commitment to achieve them. It's time to incorporate positive thought, a positive mindset, and positive actions into every day. We must wake up with the intention to move in a positive direction and believe in the direction we are moving. We will start with seven days of positive affirmations around achieving our goals. Each day for the next seven days, we will write three affirmations associated with achieving our dreams on a sticky note and post them in a different spot you will see throughout your day. For example, "I have the potential to achieve my dreams," "I am a courageous person who doesn't live in fear," and "I will succeed in the face of adversity." At the end of 7 days, you will have 21 affirmations to use as weapons against self-doubt, self-deception, self-judgment, and irrational thoughts. Belief in yourself is the beginning of a miraculous ride toward contentment and success. Let's do this. I believe in you.

"Never give up on what you really want to do. The person with big dreams is more powerful than the one with all the facts."—Albert Einstein.

Letting GO Day 7

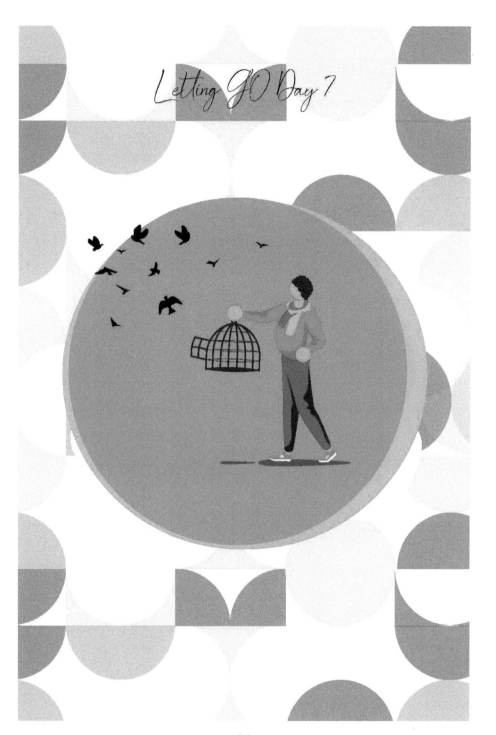

Letting Go – Day 7

In order to let go of something, we first must identify what we are holding onto. The thought of letting go of anything may create a range of emotions for some of us. This is perfect! Emotions and feelings are motivators for change, and with change comes an opportunity to produce positive experiences. If you are the person who is always telling the people close to you, "I don't have control issues", you probably need this exercise the most. Some of us are fixated on controlling all aspects of the world around us, and others are holding onto resentments, beliefs, experiences, and ideas that serve us no purpose. Steve Maraboli explained, "Incredible change happens in your life when you decide to take control of what you do have power over instead of craving control over what you don't." Today can be another opportunity to lighten our load and remove some more of those rocks we carry around for no reason.

Today's intention is to identify three things we want to potentially let go of. You don't have to release them today. This is just your commitment to yourself and the universe that these people, things, or ideas no longer serve us, and we are ready to let them go. Exposing negativity will die in the light, and our opportunity to experience positivity and serenity increases.

1.) _____

2.) _____

3.) _____

Freedom begins with admittance there is a need to let go. Unbelievable positivity is produced when we completely let go. Letting go isn't always comfortable, but growth comes when we are courageous enough to get uncomfortable. I believe in you and encourage you to become willing to release your grip on the things holding you back. Let's let go together!

"There is no growth in the comfort zone, there is no comfort in the growth zone."

– Will Linssen

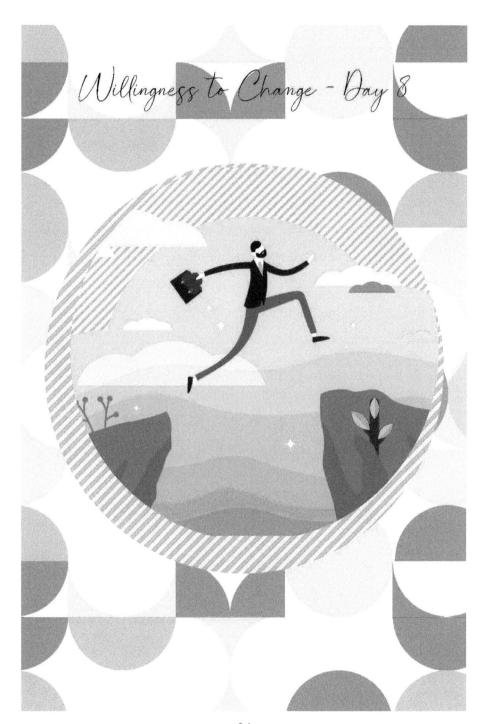

Willingness to Change – Day 8

Our ability to experience change and a more positive lifestyle is directly proportionate to our level of willingness. Wouldn't it be great if everything in life was just given to us, and we didn't have to work for anything? Endless amounts of money and material possessions just showed up on our doorstep daily, and we woke up every day in an extremely joyful mood. News flash…That movie is debuting at your local movie theater this weekend, and now we will get back to our regular scheduled programming. A life of joy, success, and stability requires the willingness to make changes in our lives. Willingness is the key to change, and without it, we will find ourselves in the same vicious cycle we have always been in. They say insanity is doing the same thing over and over again and expecting different results. The true definition of insanity is doing the same thing repeatedly, knowing exactly what is going to happen, and doing it anyway. Bill Crawford stated, "Sometimes our ability to accept what we can't change is tied to our willingness to change what we can."

We tend to get stuck in a cycle of "this is as good as it gets" or "My life will always be this way." Becoming willing to accept change opens the door to a manifestation of beauty we never believed possible. We must direct our focus to the things we have control over and not people, places, and things outside of ourselves. Exerting energy in these arenas produces no fruit and sucks from our spirit. Wasted energy depletes us of our own willingness to make changes.

Today we will set our intentions to become willing to change. Our current narrative and negative self-talk can lead to a negative mindset. This negative mindset has the potential to lead to a lack of willingness. In order to change our perception of ourselves and our ability to change, we must begin to speak love and light into our lives. Below we will complete an "I am willing to" practice and establish five things we are willing to change or let go of.

1.) I am willing to

_____

2.) I am willing to

_____

3.) I am willing to

_____

4.) I am willing to

_____

5.) I am willing to

_____

Throughout the book we will have several opportunities to implement these changes in our lives. Today we are solely focused on establishing what we are willing to change. As we move forward, we will benefit from returning to this list on a regular basis and speaking these out loud to ourselves. This will lead to positive thoughts and feelings. When we think positively, and feel positive, we become willing to act positive. This is the start of a beautiful journey, and I am excited about what the future holds for you.

"If you are willing to change your thinking, you can change your feelings. If you can change your feelings, you can change your actions. And changing your actions, based on good thinking, can change your life." –John C. Maxwell

Boundaries—Day 9

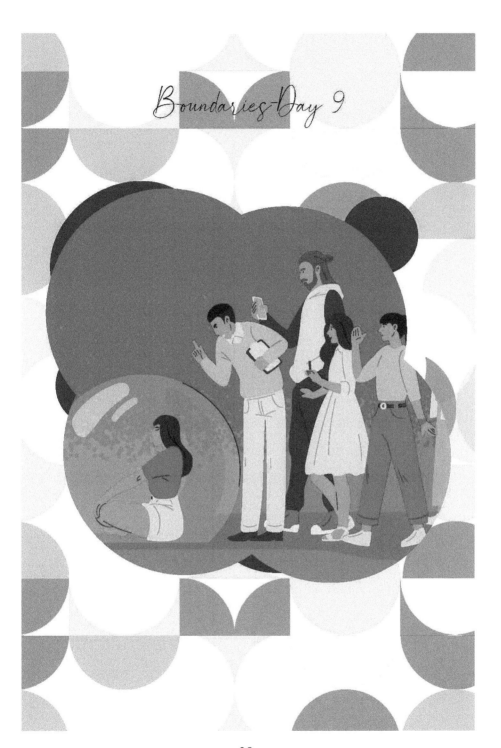

Boundaries – Day 9

When we lack boundaries, we lack self-respect and the respect of others. Our boundaries, or our lack of them, are directly correlated to our past experiences. From a young age, our environment begins to influence our understanding of healthy boundaries. It doesn't matter if we grow up in a house filled with love, connection, and support. Or a house filled with toxicity, violence, abuse, disconnection, and control. We are all susceptible to issues with boundaries. If you land in one of these categories or somewhere in the middle, there are opportunities for change. We must first identify how our unhealthy boundaries impact us and then move toward positive action.

Healthy boundaries protect us from negative physical contact, negative verbal interactions, and maintain a safe personal space. It is equally as important we utilize boundaries to keep us in, as it is to keep others at a healthy distance. Some of us take it a step further and establish walls. These are developed over time as a defense mechanism to keep us safe in situations that create danger. Walls keep us from being hurt, experiencing pain, avoiding feelings, and getting uncomfortable. Avoidance manifests into complacency and impacts our maturation process through all aspects of life. These walls inhibit us from experiencing love, connection, empathy, gratitude, and compassion. All of which we need to live positive and fulfilling lives. Our feelings and pain are looked at to be negative, but actually they create character, emotional maturity, and growth. Edwin Louis Cole explained, "Boundaries are to protect life, not to limit pleasures."

Today we will set our intentions to identify unhealthy boundaries or walls we have established in our lives that no longer serve us. Take a few minutes to sit with yourself and use the space below to write down people, situations, or things you are struggling to have healthy boundaries with. This could be your partner, a co-worker, or a friend whose only motive for being nice is to get something in return. News flash...this isn't a reciprocal relationship, it's transactional. It could also be your inability to say no to your boss when they ask you to work outside of your regular work hours on special projects. FYI...being a good employee and a doormat are two different things.

1.) _____

2.) _____

3.) _____

Our combined intentions throughout this book help us move towards self-love, self-respect, and to find our voice. We are beginning to establish a better sense of who we are, what we are willing to accept, and the caliber of people we want to surround ourselves with. There isn't an expectation today we will miraculously speak our truths and have great boundaries, but awareness is the key to change. Exposing these areas into the universe opens the door for this change. In some cases, we may not need to say anything. Our actions may speak loud enough. The opportunities to provoke change will arise. Just be patient, and follow your heart. The truth can be insulting, but it is still our truth. And remember, "No" is a full sentence. I believe in you....Lets do this!

"We can say what we need to say. We can gently, but assertively, speak our mind. We do not need to be judgmental, tactless, blaming or cruel when we speak our truths."

- Melody Beattie

Love-Day 10

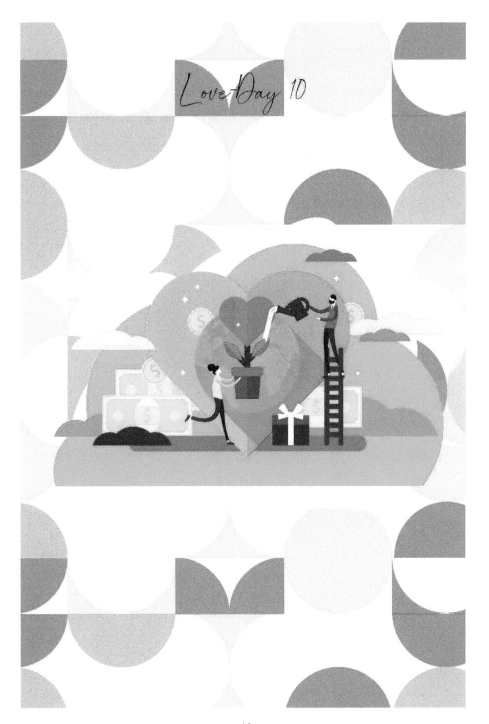

Love – Day 10

Love is such a powerful and scary word. Some of us have a hard time showing it, and others have a hard time receiving it. Regardless of what category you fall under, we all need it. We are all born as pristine vehicles with no scratches, no dents, dings, or issues. As we grow and move through different stages of the development process, we are exposed to situations and pain that consequently bang up a fender, crack our windshield, cause a tire to go flat, or blow our engine completely. If you have no interest in cars, this metaphor may not make sense to you, but hold onto the wheel…the punch line is coming. Some of us show up at this very moment in our lives with no gas left in the tank or on blocks with no hope of ever restoring our vehicle (ourselves) back to what it once was. The process begins with loving ourselves enough to do the work to create change and begin the restoration process. As we begin to embark on a journey of self-love, the capacity to experience love for others and receive it in return, will manifest in our lives. Paul McCartney said it himself, "All you need is love". It must be true.

Today is the day to set our intention to focus on loving ourselves and extending love to others. First, grab a sticky note and write I love you followed by your name. Stick this somewhere you will see throughout the day. Every time you see it, read it out loud and proud. Now in the space provided below, write three positive affirmations. For example, I am worthy of love and belonging!

1.) _____

2.) _____

3.) _____

You will return to these three affirmations throughout the day when you get into that **Stinking Thinking!**

For those who have a hard time showing themselves love, that exercise may have been AWKWARD! For those who have a hard time showing others love….well, this could make you cringe a little. It's simple but will have a significant impact on you and others. Just pick up the phone and call, send a text, or send an IM to 5 people and tell them you love them. That's it! The next gift comes with reciprocity, as we begin to receive the love in return. I love you and believe in you. Let's go spread some love!

"The love we give away is the only love we keep."

--Elbert Hubbard

Open-minded-Day 11

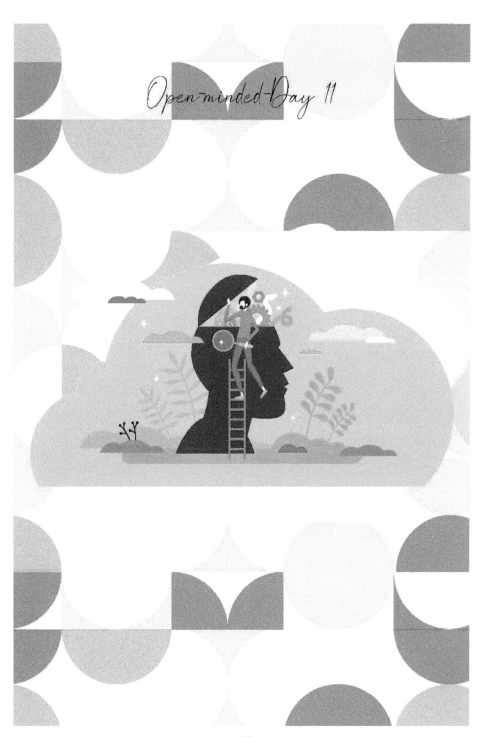

Open-minded – Day 11

Maintaining a state of open-mindedness allows change to occur. Being closed-minded increases our chances of negative thoughts, negative perspectives, and a negative lifestyle. We spend our entire lives being influenced by different ideas through our experiences and interactions. When we are young, we embrace what our elders say as the truth and follow their lead. As we get older, we begin to see things through our own set of lenses, and our perspective becomes more ridged. The combination of our environment growing up and our experiences as adults create a belief system inside us that we believe to be the truth, the whole truth, and nothing but the truth.

Our ridged and skewed perception of things will create barriers between us and the opportunity for positive change. In order to create change in our lives, we need to remain open-minded to other ideas and people's perspectives. We are faced with a dilemma when we pass judgment on people because their ideas or beliefs are different than ours. This will instantly negate our opportunity to learn from them. We must see past our judgment and move to a place of acceptance if we want to reap the benefits of what others have to offer.

"Remember a closed mind is like a closed parachute. It is of no use, and a big burden on your back!" - Abhishek Thakore

Today we will set our intentions to become more open-minded. In order for this to take place, we must become willing to hear others out and see things from a different perspective. We will begin with a brief narrative centered around open-mindedness. Feel free to create your own in the space provided, but there is an example for you below. Repeat the narrative at least five times right now.

Today I will focus on opening myself and my mind up to new ideas. I will not pass judgment on others because their ideas and beliefs are different than mine. I want to grow, change, and experience new things. I know this requires me to have an open mind.

Your own narrative;

_____

_____

_____

_____

_____

When we provide our brains with new information, it opens us up to new ideas. We can add this narrative to our tool belt and go back to it as we move forward on this journey of producing positivity. Now we will establish 3 things we would like to become more open-minded too. This will differ from person to person. Add these to the space provided below.

1.) _____

2.) _____

3.) _____

As always, awareness is the key to change, and when we bring things to light, we open the door for a new perspective. In the coming days, these things we have established will present themselves in our lives and provide us with the opportunity to be open-minded. When this occurs, remember the narrative and our objective through this process is to produce positivity in our lives. Changes in our perspective may be uncomfortable, but the end results could revolutionize our existence. I believe in you and your ability to open your mind.

"The humility to learn from one and all and keeping an open mind, is the hallmark of the truly great." –The Indian Journal of Adult Education

Commitment-Day 12

Commitment – Day 12

We all lack follow-through at times, and when we fall short, we are quick to judge ourselves. We look at failure as a bad thing, and as we move through life, it creates a lack of confidence inside our spirit. We have the best of intentions to complete tasks but talk ourselves out of things at the last minute. In other instances, we commit to things "We will do tomorrow". Tomorrow comes, nothing gets done, and we make a commitment to do the same thing again "tomorrow". Unfortunately, the task never gets done. Over time the vicious cycle of shame and guilt creates core beliefs of "I am a failure", "I will never be good enough", "I can't do this", or "I will never change". We start to believe we will never be able to follow through and get that last piece of the puzzle in place. Change in behavior creates change in our beliefs.

Today we set our intentions to identify and follow through on three simple commitments. No one is asking you to run a marathon, but if you want to, that's great. There are no expectations you commit to changing the world today, but if your heart desires that, please go for it. These are things you can do today no matter what! Ultimately, leading to us experiencing a sense of accomplishment. In order to start to change to a more positive thought pattern, we must begin to behave more positively. When we have a positive experience, we create a new reference point and open up new neuropathways in our brains. What is a neuropathway you ask...google it! Let's do this.

Below, you will find three lines to write down your commitments.

1._____
2._____
3._____

That wasn't all that hard. Now the work begins. I believe in you. Lets go out and follow through on these commitments like your life depends on it. Maybe it does! Have a beautiful day, and embrace the fruits of your labor.

"A change is brought about because ordinary people do extraordinary things."

\- Barack Obama

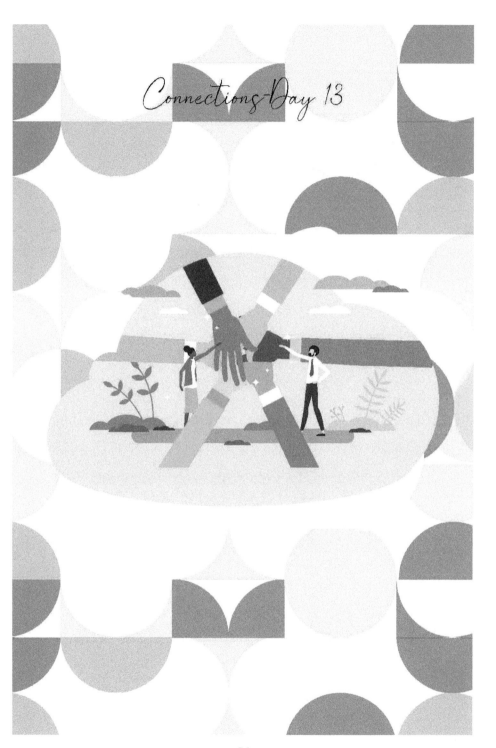

Connections–Day 13

Connections – Day 13

Finding genuine connections to people, places, and things that enrich our lives is essential to producing positivity in our spirits. The reality is we all have experiences in the past that have shifted our perspectives in a negative direction. This differs from person to person and from one stage of life to the next. When we are young and in school, it is natural for us to feel the need to be liked by a large group of our peers, and if we aren't, we identify ourselves as "the outcast". We will find ourselves on the outside looking in when we don't feel we fit into the box society says we should. We may also feel disconnected due to not getting invited to lunch with the team at work, not getting picked to play on a sports team, being ghosted after dating for a while, someone not responding to an email, or even a friend not tagging us in a social media post. These are a few of potentially millions of examples of things that create a disconnection between us and the world around us. John Lennon said, "You may say I'm a dreamer, but I'm not the only one. I hope someday you'll join us. And the world will live as one." Quit dreaming about being on the inside of the circle, and jump in. Today is the day.

Several other positive-producing principles and practices in this book will help create a connection for you. Today's intention is to begin believing we are worthy of genuine connections. The word "Genuine" is an essential part of this exercise because those of us who have spent our whole lives "being the cool kid" actually only have a few genuine connections. And those of us who have experienced trauma or been the "outcast" don't believe we are worthy of anything genuine. Below is a space for us to establish a positive narrative focused on manifesting genuine positive connections in our life. Here is an example:

- I am an amazing, authentic, and awesome human being who is worthy of genuine love and connection.

Now it's your turn to develop a sentence or two you can speak into existence throughout the day and for the days to come. What we speak about, we can bring about, and positivity is what we are producing. Remain mindful of this sentence throughout the day, and allow it to become a mainstay in your pattern of thought.

1._____

_____

There are no guarantees you will immediately create a sense of connection through this exercise, but with continued practice of positive self-talk, our perception of ourselves and the world around us will change. As our perception changes, our connections will change. We experience connection by believing we are worthy of it. You are worthy of it, and you deserve it. Let's get connected.

"We are like islands in the sea, separate on the surface but connected in the deep." - William James

Acceptance-Day 14

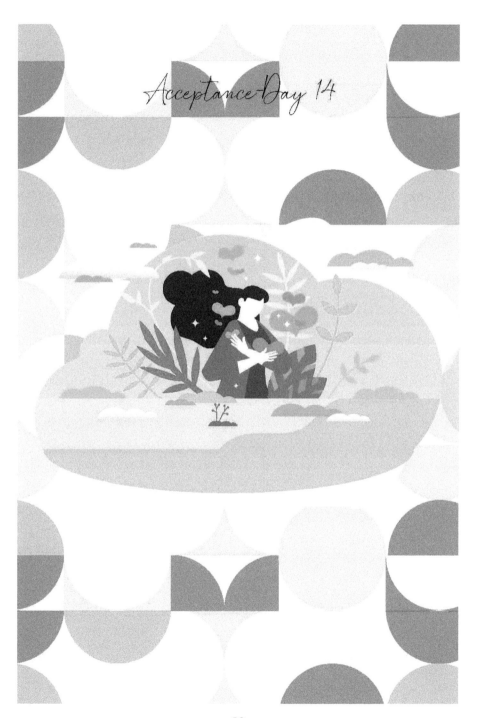

Acceptance – Day 14

Today we set out with the intention to practice acceptance in all areas of our life. Acceptance isn't a quality that comes naturally to many of us. Nor is it easy to be okay with things that don't go our way. A wise man Jimmy Isch once said, "Acceptance is the fertile soil from which other spiritual principles grow. I can't be grateful for something until I accept it. I can't truly love someone until I accept them as they are. I can't have faith in something until I first accept it." This perspective is so profoundly positive and a shift in this direction could be life changing.

We are faced with a dilemma when we try to grow things in unfertile ground. Forcing our beliefs and imposing our will on people, places, and things is similar to planting flowers in concrete. Today is the day we begin our new practice of acceptance and cultivate positivity and principles into our soil. This will provide a space for beautiful and fruitful growth to occur.

Below are a few examples of narratives we can use when we find ourselves in a negative internal dialogue regarding the world around us.

- I will accept (enter name here) right where they are at, and not where I expect them to be.

- I don't agree with this, but it will work out just fine.

Now it is your turn to establish three statements to add to your tool belt you can use to accept things you inherently have a hard time accepting.

1.) _____

_____

2.) _____

_____

3.) _____

_____

Acceptance is the key to change, and today we are ready to change. Let's do this, I believe in you.

"We cannot become what we want by remaining what we are."

– Max Depree

Service-Day 15

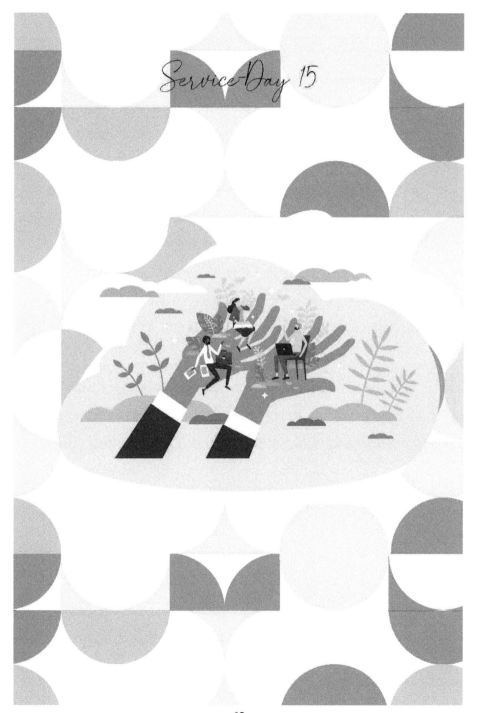

Service – Day 15

When we talk about service in this book, we aren't talking about "can you hear me now" or "can I please get another glass of soda." The service identified here is the kind we do to help and encourage others. Humans tend to be self-centered, self-absorbed, and selfish. We live in a world more focused on competing and collecting than compassion and giving. Many of us claim not to have time to give of ourselves to others because we have developed beliefs like "there aren't enough hours in the day" or "my time is precious." Statements like this breed self-centeredness and drive a wedge between us and the world. This wedge inhibits our ability to experience the therapeutic value we receive when we are of service to others.

Something as simple as a hello in the grocery store or words of encouragement to a friend, family member, or co-worker is a form of service. Mother Theresa stated, "Kind words can be short and easy to speak, but their echoes are truly endless." The ripple effect of positivity we send out is truly endless and has the potential to inspire others to serve as well. There are more formal forms of service everywhere around us. Our communities and those living in them need us. There are hundreds of agencies, non-profits, groups, churches, etc., that need our help. Service to others provides us with purpose, connection, and interaction. All of which create a release of feel-good chemicals in the brain. I like to feel good. I bet you do too!

Today we set our intentions to be more selfless and less selfish. We will intentionally speak love and kindness into everyone we come in contact with throughout the day. If a simple hello is the best you can do, great. I challenge you to be a little riskier and dive off the surface when engaging with others. What do you have to lose? Below you will find a few examples of ideas you could say.

- Your outfit looks amazing today.

- Nice shoes!

- I appreciate what you bring to the team in the office, and I am grateful for you.

- Our marriage means the world to me, and I am blessed to be on this journey with you.

- Thank you for always being such a good friend.

We are encouraged to be authentic and come from a place of love and kindness when engaging with the world. It serves us no purpose if we don't mean what we say. People will see right through us, and our words will have little to no impact. More importantly, we will know we are being fake. We are striving to be our true, authentic, and positive self through this process. This will create positivity.

Now we will develop a list of three different volunteer opportunities we are interested in. If you are already volunteering in the community or are of service, use this space to establish ways to enhance what you are already doing.

1.) _____

2.) _____

3.) _____

This world is a better place because we are in it, and each act of service we do today increases the impact we have. Be the change you want to see and spread that positivity….I believe in you.

"Those who are the happiest are those who do the most for others"

—Booker T. Washington

Reciprocity-Day 16

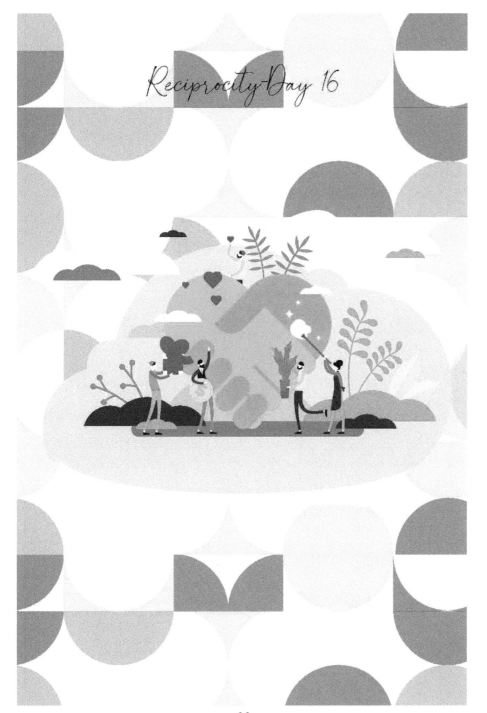

Reciprocity – Day 16

In order to receive good things in the world, we must be willing to give. What do I give, you may ask? We give ourselves, our time, our love, and our attention. We give our hearts to others, a non-judgmental ear, a safe space, or our experience. When we give these things away, we increase our chances of producing positivity. Reciprocity from a social aspect is similar to the law of attraction and the belief that what we give away, we will receive in return. Relationships built on authenticity, love, connection, and vulnerability are breeding grounds for reciprocity. They are mutually beneficial, and we grow stronger foundations because we are pouring into each other and not constantly taking away. Our lives begin to manifest into beautiful works of art, and the interweaving of the tapestry connects our spirits together. We are dependent on others to feel safe and loved. The principle of reciprocity provides a consistent flow of energy back and forth between us and those around us.

"The basis of social relationships is reciprocity: if you cooperate with others, others will cooperate with you." - Carroll Quigley

Our intentions should never be to do good things with the expectation of receiving good things in return. We set our intentions to serve, love, be kind, connect, and be authentic each day because it is the right thing to do. People will fall short, and if we have expectations, we will be let down consistently. Acceptance of people's shortcomings allows us to continue to shine brightness in the presence of darkness. If we give into the temptation to reciprocate negativity, we will surely receive it in return. People will meet us with the same energy we exude.

Today we will set our intention to shine bright in all of our affairs. Principles are easy to practice and apply when things are going great. It's in those challenging times, with challenging people, we must stay strong and centered. Let's start with a little breathwork meditation. If you are brand new to meditation don't worry. We are simply breathing and counting. Find a quiet, comfortable place and begin with 10 deep breaths in through your nose and out through your nose. Each breath in and out is one count. As you transition into your eleventh breath sequence, start to visualize breathing in positivity on your in-breath and negativity out on your out-breath. Continue with this breath cycle and visualization for as long as you like. Our central nervous system is now calming and in a restful state. This may not last all day, and challenging situations may create a fight-or-flight response inside of us. If this occurs, take a few minutes to return to your breath, and once again, breathe in positivity and out negativity. Remaining peaceful and centered throughout the day keeps the door open for the positive flow of energy to be reciprocated.

Be intentional today when opportunities arise to share your heart, positive energy, or love. This exchange between us and the world creates building blocks to positivity. The feel-good emotions we invoke inside of our spirit by remaining centered and practicing reciprocity will create a foundation we are proud to stand on. Lets go do this....I believe in you!

"Abundance is a dance with reciprocity-what we can give, what we can share, and what we receive in the process" - Terry Tempest Williams

Self-Care Day 17

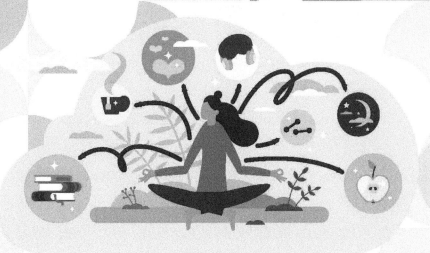

Self-Care – Day 17

The importance of self-care can be minimized at times due to our inability to make ourselves important. Caring for others is what we are supposed to do, right? To some extent this is true, but when our needs aren't met, or even worse, our mental, physical, emotional, and spiritual health is suffering, we need to make some changes. Many of us fall into the trap of fixing others to avoid looking at the areas in our own lives that need work. Some of us put so much emphasis on trying to fix, manage, and control everyone around us, that we haven't taken the time to look in the mirror for many years. There are others who are experiencing extremely low self-esteem due to negative core beliefs, and we lack the ability to love ourselves enough to make self-care important. Regardless of what category you may fall into, it's okay, you are not alone. If you were to ask most people in the world, how is your self-care? They would almost always respond, "it could be better."

We didn't get to the point we are at overnight, and it will take some time to incorporate a regular self-care routine into our daily practice. We need to be patient and compassionate with ourselves through the process. The identification of a need for change is the beginning of self-love. Self-care is impossible if we are incapable or unwilling to love ourselves. Our body, mind, and spirit are our biggest resources, and we must invest in them. Some of us are lacking in one of these areas, and others need adjustments in all areas.

"With every act of self-care your authentic self gets stronger, and the critical, fearful mind gets weaker. Every act of self-care is a powerful declaration: I am on my side, I am on my side, each day I am more on my own side." – Susan Weiss Berry

Today we set our intentions to increase our self-care. Some of us may have a routine that solely needs some adjustments, and others may need a full overhaul. We can start with simple tasks such as spending time each day sitting in a quiet place in self-reflection. Taking a 15-minute walk around the neighborhood by ourselves. Treating ourselves to a manicure or a pedicure is a wonderful act of self-care. Yes, fellas, men do this too! We can incorporate time in each day to read self-help or inspirational material that will increase our overall spiritual, mental, and emotional conditioning. Taking ourselves out for a nice dinner is magical. Increasing our exercise routine or making some adjustments to our eating habits can make monumental changes in how we feel about ourselves. These are just ideas to provoke thought, and the possibilities are endless.

First, we will establish two self-care activities we are going to do today. These are things you don't normally do, but you can complete them today regardless of what other things may seem to be a priority. Remember, you are your greatest resource. Add these in the space provided.

1.) _____

2.) _____

Now we will establish two things per week we will begin to incorporate into our daily living on a consistent basis over the next three weeks. We will slowly increase and add two activities a week until we have successfully added six total new self-care activities.

Week 1:

1.) _____

2.) _____

Week 2:

1.) _____

2.) _____

Week 3:

1.) _____

2.) _____

Statistics show half of the things will become a regular part of our lives after 60 days. And over the course of 6 months, we will become complacent and be left with one or two of the activities we added. Some may look at this as a bad thing, but if every six months we add a couple of self-care activities to our lives, in five years we will be in a much better place. Every journey starts with one step, and over time we will begin to experience returns on our investment in ourselves. I believe in you. Today is the day you increase your belief and love in yourself.

"When you recover or discover something that nourishes your soul and brings joy, care enough about yourself to make room for it in your life." – Jean Shinoda Bolen

Gratitude-Day 18

Gratitude – Day 18

Gratitude is a gift we can share with the world. We spend a large portion of life seeking opportunities and things to make us happy. True happiness doesn't come from the pursuit of being happy, but from intentionally being grateful. We can have everything we ever dreamed of, fancy cars, a big house, a surplus of money, private jets, and not be happy. If by chance you have a private jet and aren't happy, this book is truly meant for you. Seriously though, why is it we put so much emphasis on having things to create happiness? As established previously, society has been conditioning us to think in this way since we were born. Commercials, social media, news, magazines, family members, our parents, and our peers impose beliefs on us that without things, we won't be happy. We are a society focused so much on competition and getting more stuff, we don't take any time being grateful for the things and beautiful people we already have. Christiane Northrup states, "Feeling grateful or appreciative of someone or something in your life actually attracts more of the things that you appreciate and value into your life." Gratitude is the path to happiness, joy, peace, and serenity. This path will create positivity in our lives and those around us.

Today we will set our intentions on identifying things we are grateful for and practice gratefulness. There are several different methods or practices we can implement into our daily routine. We can journal daily on gratitude, verbalize a gratitude list, write one down, meditate on gratitude, share with others how grateful we are they are in our lives, and also share our gratitude through our actions. These are methods designed to increase gratitude and ultimately attract more of the things we value and appreciate into our lives. When identifying things we are grateful for, we want to focus on the things we were given or gifts we have received. Not solely on material possessions or wealth. These things may make us comfortable but don't guarantee happiness. For example:

I am grateful for the beating of my heart, the breath in my lungs, and the opportunity to have a positive impact on the world today.

First, we will establish a gratitude list with 5 things we are grateful for.

1.) _____

2.) _____

3.) _____

4.) _____

5.) _____

Now we will set our intentions to go out and share our gratitude with others through our actions. We have been building up to this point throughout the book. Today we will bring several components together and intentionally serve others, spread positivity, practice love, be authentic, and create connections.

"I don't have to chase extraordinary moments to find happiness – it's right in front of me if I'm paying attention and practicing gratitude."– Brene Brown

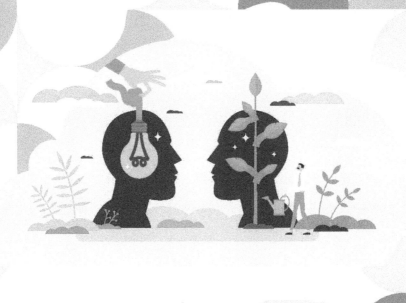

Inspired by Relationships – Day 19

We will find inspiration from our relationships if we surround ourselves with inspiring people. From birth we are dependent on people to help us navigate life, inspire us, and help us survive. Dating back thousands of years, we have drawn strength from the people in our tribe and are reliant on each other. Everyone brings a skill, personality trait, characteristics, and contribution to the table. Diversity eliminates the need for anyone to be an expert at everything. Accepting our role and embracing our strengths and limitations is key to feeling secure in our relationships. As children, we have an innate need to compete with our siblings, cousins, friends, and peers. This competition creates a drive within us to be better, but in contrast, it can lead to comparison and insecurity. Carl Jung wrote, "The meeting of two personalities is like the contact of two chemical substances: if there is any reaction, both are transformed." This reaction Jung speaks of has the potential to create inspiration and positivity in the relationship if we embrace our individuality.

We must move away from comparison, envy, and jealousy when those around us are experiencing victory. This drives a wedge between us and the benefits of hope and inspiration we will feel. Surrounding ourselves with people on a similar path increases our opportunity to move in the direction we want to go. Other people's successes in life are confirmation we can achieve the same things. If the people in our lives aren't our biggest fans, we must find different people. On the flip side, we have a responsibility to be cheerleaders too. *"For beautiful eyes, look for the good in others; for beautiful lips, speak only words of kindness; and for poise, walk with the knowledge that you are never alone."*— Audrey Hepburn.

Today we set out with the intention to inspire those who inspire us. Our ability to do this is directly proportionate to our current perception of who we are and our level of self-love. We will take a couple of minutes to do some verbal positive affirmation work. The hope is by this point in our process of producing positivity in our lives, we are using the tools provided. Daily positive affirmations are key to increased self-acceptance and self-love. Below is a short affirmation narrative we will read out loud at least five times in a row.

I love myself and embrace the unique qualities I bring to my relationships. I am an asset to all of the people in my life, and I am diligently working to be the best I can be. I accept my assets and my liabilities, and I wouldn't want to be anyone else.

Now we will make a list of the top five people who inspire us. These are the people who provide us with hope when we are hopeless, encouragement when we are discouraged, unconditional love when we can't love ourselves, and shine light in our darkest times.

1.) _____

2.) _____

3.) _____

4.) _____

5.) _____

Today we will break out our pom poms and cheer for these people who are always cheering for us. We can do this via phone, text, flowers, a social media post, gifts, taking them out for a meal, a large sum of money, or a simple hug and thank you. The specific activities in which we show our appreciation for them aren't as important as just doing something. Acknowledging the role these people play in our lives helps us identify and embrace the role we play in theirs. Relationships aren't about competition…. They are about inspiration. Let's do this….I believe in you.

"Success is liking yourself, liking what you do, and liking how you do it."

— Maya Angelou.

Courageous-Day 20

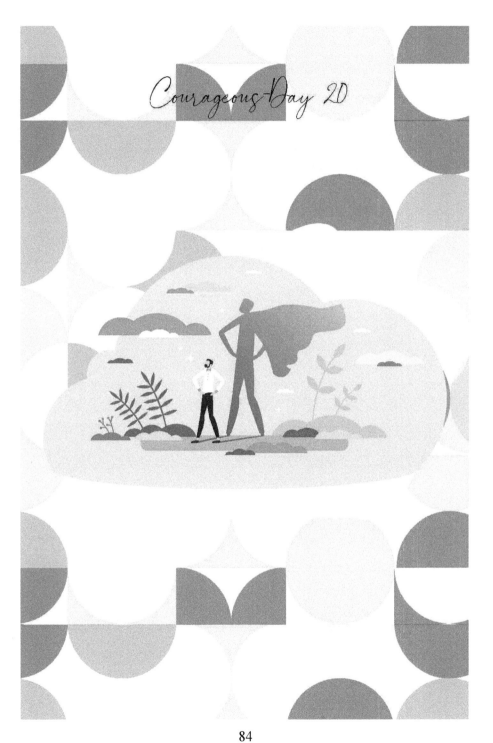

Courageous – Day 20

Courage, or the act of being courageous, comes from the belief we are capable of accomplishing things even when adversity is guaranteed. If we have experienced a history of failure and have developed the core belief, "we aren't enough", there is a probability we may lack courage. We may see ourselves as the Cowardly Lion in the Wizard of Oz or Thomas the Train before he believed he was the little engine that could. The environment we grow up in will also dictate how courageous we are. We have a better chance of growing up with confidence and courage if we witness those around us exemplifying these qualities. From birth, we are dependent on people to guide us, encourage us, and pour love into us. The role models in our lives are instrumental in nurturing strong beliefs into us about our abilities, talents, and potential. It is through encouragement; we develop the ability to be courageous. As we transition into adulthood, we remain dependent on outside sources to encourage us, but our true source of strength comes from within. We become our biggest cheerleaders, and with the correct internal dialogue, we can walk through the most challenging events like a warrior on Braveheart. John Wayne said it perfectly, "Courage is being scared to death and saddling up anyway."

There is a wide variable in which we define the level of courage needed to put forth depending on the seriousness of the situation. Skydiving for the first time and asking someone for help are both courageous acts, but the level of courage may differ. Walking through both situations creates new positive reference points for us and will increase our belief in ourselves. Our brain needs new information in order to begin the rewiring process from consistent self-doubt to self-confidence. We have focused our attention on negative aspects of our character for long enough.

"Only passions, great passions can elevate the soul to do great things."

- Denis Diderot

Today we will set our intention to be courageous and identify different situations where we practice courage. We will begin with a short positive affirmation narrative focused on courage and confidence. We can develop our own or repeat the one provided. Repeat this at least five times out loud while looking in the mirror.

I am a powerful human being who is capable of walking through any discomfort, pain, challenges, or fear I may face today. I am confident, strong-willed, and courageous. I will rise up because I can.

Now we will set out in search of opportunities to be courageous. It is imperative we identify all of them and not minimize any act of courage. In the space below, we will list all the times we were courageous. The details of the event are not as important as simply writing them down. Some of us may have the ability to write throughout the day, and others may utilize the evening as a time for reflection and writing. Both will work just fine. The important thing is we write. More space is available in the book if needed. Magic happens when we see the words come alive on the page in front of us. Confidence can be created by this simple act of identification of the courage with which we practiced. Let's be courageous today...I believe in you.

"Courage is not the absence of fear, but the triumph over it. The brave man is not he who does not feel afraid, but he who conquers that fear."

—Nelson Mandela

Authenticity Day 21

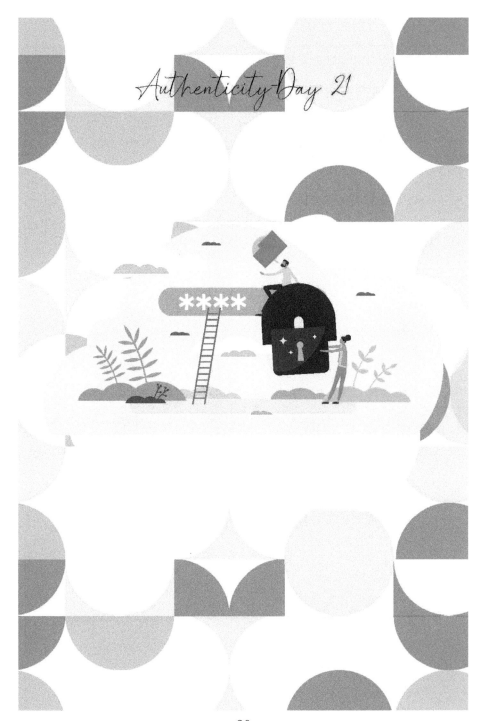

Authenticity – Day 21

The true version of ourselves is best represented when we are authentic. Over time we all develop masks that protect us from judgment, criticism, accountability, and danger. These masks become a part of us, but they aren't who we truly are at the core. The longer and more frequently we wear them, the more comfortable they become. This creates a belief inside of us we aren't okay without them, and we spend a lot of energy suiting up to be someone each day we weren't created to be. The energy we spend doing this can be draining, suffocating, and overwhelming. If you identify with this, you are not alone. The world wants to know the true version of who we are, and for us to experience the freedom available by being authentic. If by chance you wear a Halloween mask around to create joy and positivity, by all means, keep rocking it. We love to laugh. We are solely focused on the metaphorical ones here.

Our masks protect us, but they also separate us from all the meaningful components of life. Dan Tibbits shared, "Authenticity starts with self-honesty and is my path to intimacy. When I show up with an image of myself, everyone else just gets a mirage. To be connected I need to be real. It opens the door both ways for empathy, and through that door I end up truly free and in love."

Today we will begin by setting our intention to remove one mask we regularly wear. For example, the "tough guy/gal" mask. This is regularly worn by people who are experiencing emotional pain on the inside but keep a stoic, well-put-together appearance on the outside. Then there are those of us who are insecure and anxious around people. Instead of being honest and authentic, we put on the "I am a loner" mask, and avoid society like the plague. Consequently, this mask builds walls around us and shields us from what we truly want, social connection.

All we have to do today is identify the one mask we want to wear less and add it into the space provided.

"I identify I wear the _____ mask on a daily basis, and today I proclaim this mask must go." Now read the statement above out loud 5 times to yourself.

This is the start of a restoration process towards becoming the person you were created to be and not the person you invented. Establishing this in writing opens up an opportunity for change. Self-awareness is the key to change, and it is on you to avoid putting this mask on as often. In order to become more comfortable with the true you, you will need new experiences without the mask. We must get uncomfortable in order to get comfortable, and today is the day we start this journey. I believe in you, and it is time you develop an authentic relationship with yourself.

"Only the truth of who you are, if realized, will set you free."

– Eckhart Tolle.

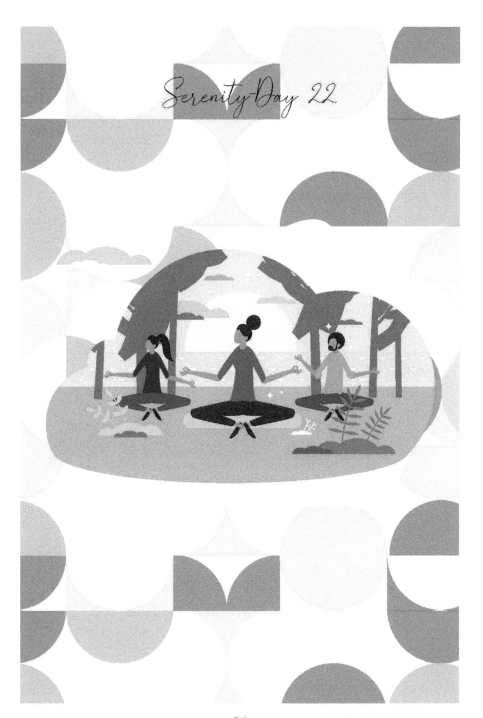

Serenity-Day 22

Serenity – Day 22

Serenity is something we all deserve to experience, but many of us continuously live in chaos. Our hearts are constantly in conflict with our minds, and we feel overwhelmed. Work, kids, relationships, politics, world conflict, interpersonal challenges, financial struggles, health concerns, and an assortment of other life events create a dis-ease in our spirit. At times we find ourselves holding on by the seat of our pants and not enjoying the moments. Worry, doubt, fear, shame, guilt, and regret consume us. We spend more time living in the past and the future than we do in the present. Ruminating in the past can drive depression, and staying fixated on the future can create anxiety. Neither of which is in congruence with serenity.

"Every breath we take, every step we make, can be filled with joy, peace, and serenity."

– Thich Nhat Hanh

Today we will set our intentions to focus solely on the present moment, and not the past or future. At times throughout the day, you may find yourself pulling out your crystal ball and predicting your future. Unless you are a fortune teller, these are skills you don't possess. At other moments you may find yourself fixated on those "shoulda," "woulda," and "coulda" moments from years past. It's doubtful you have a time travel machine, and NASA has no plans of making one. Crystal balls and time machines may seem like great tools, but gratitude, mindfulness, and acceptance are keys to serenity.

First, we will establish three things we are grateful for today. It is important with this gratitude list we stay focused on the events, gifts, people, or things of the present. Not yesterday or tomorrow...today. This helps condition our minds to live more in the present moment.

1.) _____

2.) _____

3.) _____

Second, we will take a few minutes to practice mindfulness and sit with our thoughts, feelings, and emotions. Find some calming music or nature sounds on the electronic device of your choice and let it play softly in the background. When we find ourselves wandering to the past or future, just gently bring yourself back to this moment and the three things, we are grateful for today.

Lastly, we will recite the serenity prayer three times out loud. If you have challenges with the word God or have a different belief system, please insert whatever definition is comfortable for you.

"God grant me the serenity to accept the things I cannot change, the courage to change the things I can, and the wisdom to know the difference."

Gratitude, mindfulness, and the serenity prayer are tools we can come back to throughout the day or days to come when we become consumed with racing thoughts of the future or rumination of the past. You deserve freedom, peace, positivity, and serenity. It's free for the taking, now go get it. I believe in you.

"Remember that wherever your heart is, there you will find your treasure."

--Paulo Coelho

Limitless Horizons-Day 23

Limitless Horizons – Day 23

Our potential to reach new limits and a life of increased positivity is possible by increasing our investment in ourselves. Our belief system dictates the path we take in life. If we believe we have reached a ceiling and there isn't anything left for us to achieve on the horizon, we will lack the motivation to change. This mindset has the potential to create a plateau far below our full potential. The people we surround ourselves with will also play a significant role in our lives. If they lack the ambition to reach new heights, we may fall into this same trap. Water seeks its own level. Do you want to drown in the swamps or swim in the ocean?

Feelings of hopelessness, discontent, lethargy, stress, self-pity, boredom, envy, jealousy, comparison, and sadness don't benefit us on our journey to producing positivity. We need to dig deep into our spirits and draw from the inner piece of our being that believes we are worthy of a life far beyond our wildest dreams.

"Stay blind to any fears or limitations and open your eyes to the inexhaustible power and infinite possibilities already inside you."

\- Hiral Nagda

Today we set our intentions to set the bar higher for ourselves and begin to detach from people, places, and things that may be holding us back. We are in control of our own destinies. Setting self-defeating prophecies and holding onto negative influences are keeping us from living up to our full potential. Today that changes! We will start by establishing a short list of things we believe are holding us back in life. These could be negative friendships, drinking alcohol, binging TV shows, excessive scrolling on social media, a current romantic relationship, or a dead-end job. Below we will write down these 3-5 things.

1.)

_____

2.)

_____

3.)

_____

4.)

_____

5.)

_____

Identification of these negative influences in our lives provides us with an awareness change is needed. As we move forward on this journey, the hope is the importance of these things will decrease and other positive influences will increase. We will now bust out our sticky notes with the intent to provoke a change of thought over the coming days. On 5-10 separate sticky notes, we will establish "Power Positivity Statements." These statements, when read, inspire us to reach for new limits in our lives. For example, "I will become an author," "I am a superhero," "I am capable of things I never thought possible', "I will make a career change and follow my dreams," and "I am worthy of a better life." You can use these as examples, but please create your own. We will now place these sticky notes in different places where we will see them on a regular basis. Our car, bathroom mirror, and refrigerator are a few good places to start. Under the toilet seat is a great place if you want to get creative. By reading these with confidence when we come across them, we will begin to create a more positive perspective and belief about ourselves and our potential. I believe in you, and I am excited for you to be the person you are destined to be.

"Destiny is not a matter of chance; it is a matter of choice. It is not a thing to be waited for, it is a thing to be achieve."

- William Jennings Bryan

Tolerance Day 24

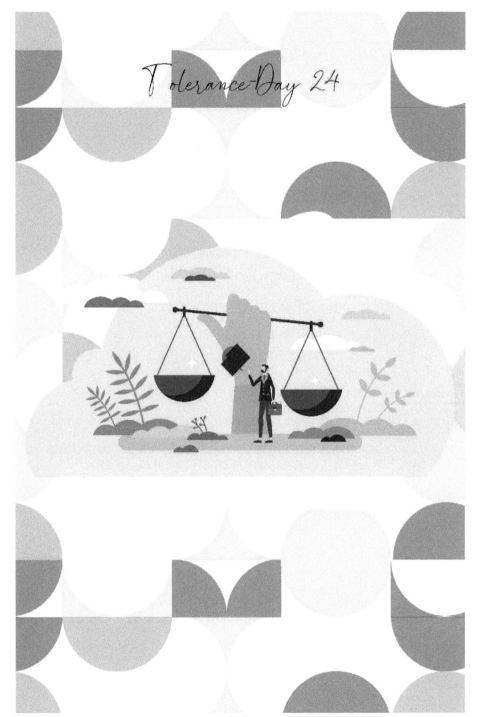

Tolerance – Day 24

Our past experiences of trauma, pain, and hurt influence our level of tolerance. In many cases, our feelings around these events are valid, but our path to positivity requires healing and acceptance. When people create pain in our lives, we believe they are out to get us or are the enemy. Dalai Lama XIV stated, "In the practice of tolerance, one's enemy is the best teacher." We are at a point in the road where we must begin to move away from our resentments, irrational beliefs, and unrealistic expectations of others, and move towards a more tolerant perspective. The diversity and unique qualities of the people we surround ourselves with provide us with a rich assortment of friends, co-workers, supervisors, family members, and associates. We need to love these individuals for their assets and their liabilities.

People are autonomous and have the freedom to make decisions that aren't always congruent with what we believe to be correct. Maintaining united and mutually beneficial relationships with these individuals is an essential component on our path to producing positivity. Unless of course, through this process you have determined someone to be toxic….by all means, they may need to go. Maintaining intolerance creates separation, poor communication, and disconnection from the people we depend on. Tony Robbins stated, "The way we communicate with others and ourselves ultimately determines the quality of our lives."

Today we will set our intentions to be more tolerant. This begins with becoming more self-aware and grounded in the present moment. We can create a more mindful state by beginning our day with a very simple breathwork meditation. If we head out into the world in a heightened state of fight or flight, we are less likely to be tolerant. Calming our mind, body, and spirit puts us in a position to embrace the world as it comes to us.

If you have your own practice, it is fine to utilize this for today's exercise. We will begin by finding a quiet, comfortable place free of any distractions. Playing some nature sounds or meditative music in the background may be beneficial. This practice is very simple and not meant to be overwhelming. It is important to remain non-judgmental of any thoughts, feelings, or sensations that may come during your meditation. The mind is designed to think, and having the expectation meditation will stop this from happening is unrealistic. We are solely focused on slowing the mind down and becoming more present in the moment.

We will begin by breathing in through the nose and out through the nose. We will count the in breath and out breath silently in our mind as we breath. In one, out two, in three, out four, in five, out six....and so on all the way until 100. If you want to continue on past 100 please do so. There is no limit on how long we can meditate. With that said, please don't miss work, the birth of a child, or an important appointment. That may be counterproductive to achieving a mindful state. We will now begin!

After completing the breathwork meditation we will come back to the moment and sit in this relaxed state focusing on what we want our interpersonal relationships and interactions with the world to be like today. We will set our intentions to maintain a state of PLUTO. We aren't talking about the dog or the planet...that may or may not be a planet. We are talking about the acronym. Patience, Love, Understanding, Tolerance, Open-mindedness

When we can apply PLUTO to our lives, we increase our opportunities to produce positivity in all areas. Today is the day we begin to move from intolerance to tolerance. I believe in you, and I am excited about what the day will bring. Let's go get it.

"Laws alone can not secure freedom of expression; in order that every man present his views without penalty there must be spirit of tolerance in the entire population."

— Albert Einstein

Wonderment-Day 25

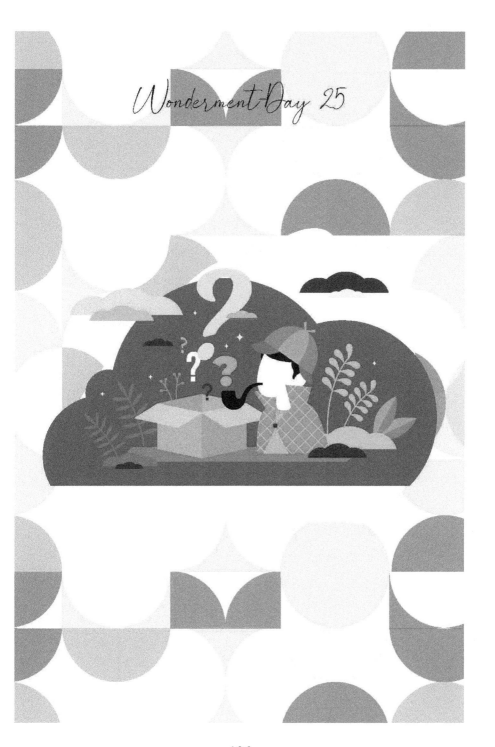

Wonderment – Day 25

What is wonderment? Wonderment is defined as a state of awe and astonishment. Remember back when we were little kids, and we experienced our first snow day, the first day we rode a bike, or the first time at an amusement park? Those are feelings of wonderment. The feeling that makes us say "AWE" or "WOW." As we grow older and experience less things for the first time, and our perception changes, we have fewer of these moments. There is a potential we may find ourselves in a mundane loop of the same thing day after day, and we no longer regularly experience wonderment. The birth of a child, a promotion, a milestone birthday, a career change, or a once-in-a-lifetime trip can all create a state of wonderment. These tend to be short-lived, and we revert back to the humdrum of life. Unfortunately, life is going 90 miles an hour, and many cultures focus more on getting onto the next "thing" and not embracing the current blessing. The reality is we don't experience fewer moments of wonderment as we grow older. We just become more consumed with the negativity and frivolous things around us, and consequently miss the moments.

"Wherever life takes us, there are always moments of wonder."

– Jimmy Carter.

Hindsight is always 20/20, and when we look back in retrospect, we can always identify moments we missed. The writing portion for today is to establish 3 moments we missed out on because we were there, but not really there. Those times when our physical body was present in the room, but our mind was trying to solve tomorrow's problems. Yes, those times. Go into as much detail as you would like, but our true intention is to raise our awareness. Awareness is the key to change, and through this act, we promote positive change.

1.)_____

_____

_____

_____

_____

2.)_____

_____

_____

_____

_____

3.)_____

_____

_____

_____

_____

We will now set our intentions on increasing our opportunities for wonderment each day moving forward. We will intentionally live more in the moment, practice mindfulness, and live in gratitude. As we continue this practice, we increase our opportunities to experience wonderment. For example, imagine yourself on train ride across the countryside in Denmark. To the citizens of Denmark, this may seem like any other train ride, but to someone traveling abroad it is a great opportunity to experience the "WOW". The sights, sounds, people, animals, architecture, waterways, bridges, tunnels, and cities along the way possess beauty. Beauty we will miss if we solely focus on getting to the last stop. We no longer have to miss the journey, because we are focused on the destination. Wonderment is all around us, let's go experience it like we are children. Today we will intentionally live in the present moment….it is a gift we will never receive again.

"Life is full of wonder. We taste in our childhood, lose it as we grow up, and if we are lucky catch the magic again in those precious moments which make life a joy."

–Jack Haas

Celebrate Everything Day 26

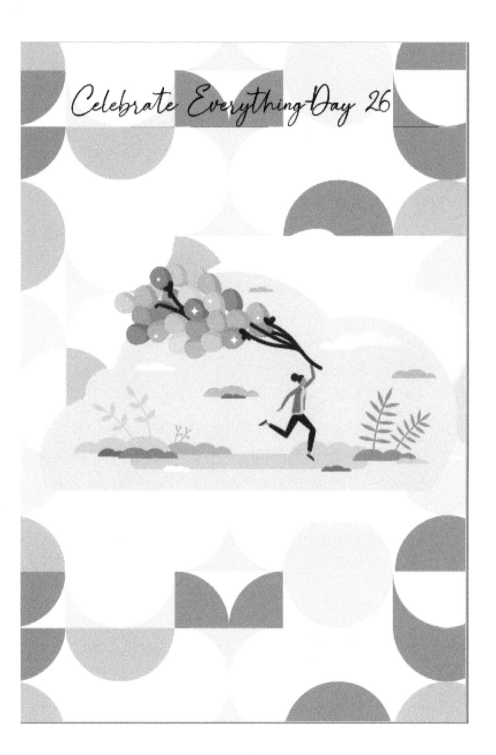

Celebrate Everything – Day 26

A positive perspective provides us with an opportunity to celebrate our accomplishments and those of the people around us. If you woke up this morning and are reading this….you won the lottery. We may not see seven zeros in our bank account, but the breath in our lungs and the beating of our hearts provide us with another opportunity to experience things we never have before. These opportunities are priceless and require celebration. Some of us have grown up in families and cultures that celebrate every phase of life. This starts shortly after conception with a gender reveal, the baby shower, the actual birth, 12 straight months of baby pictures, the first birthday…and every one after, concluding with a celebration of life when we pass away. These monumental points in our lives are worthy of being celebrated. But what about all the small things happening each day in between? Amit Ray stated, "Every day is a good day. There is something to learn, care and celebrate." When we live more in the present moment, we will bear witness to immense beauty happening all around us. This beauty is worthy of celebration.

On our path to producing positivity, we must take off our jaded glasses and begin to see life through a new set of lenses. Only celebrating the stereotypical or commercialized times in our lives robs us of the joy found day to day. Every little win should be acknowledged, validated, recognized, and celebrated. Celebration of these things may not come with balloons, confetti, or a red carpet. If these forms of celebration are appropriate…go for it. The celebration we are talking about resonates in our hearts, minds, and spirits through identification and recognition. Regardless of how big or small the win, there is an opportunity to experience gratefulness. Gratitude is our form of celebration.

Today we will set out with the intention to identify and recognize all of the wins we experience throughout the day. "Wins" are identified as anything positive, enriching, uplifting, memorable, impactful, insightful, or enjoyable. Examples of these could be holding the door open, extending love to others, practicing patience, helping a co-worker, witnessing your child excel in an activity, cleaning the house, taking 10,000 steps, reading self-help material, and so on. The potential "wins" are endless and all around us. Through identification and recognition, we will have the opportunity to increase gratitude. An attitude of gratitude leads to our overarching goal of producing positivity. The important thing is to focus on the "wins" and not "losses" or "negative things." Through this process, we are developing a new pattern of thinking.

Below you will find ample space to write down your wins throughout the day. You can start your list with "Reading this book" and "setting my intention to identify the wins." Look at us go. We are well on our way to a magical day. If possible, we will carry the book with us and take time throughout the day to list the "Wins." We will conclude our day in self-reflection and write down all the "Wins" we can remember. Let's do this...we are winners today. We will celebrate together.

_____

_____

_____

_____

_____

_____

_____

_____

_____

_____

_____

_____

_____

_____

_____

_____

_____

_____

"Celebrate who you are in your deepest heart. Love yourself and the world will love you."

— Amy Leigh Mercree

Perseverance-Day 27

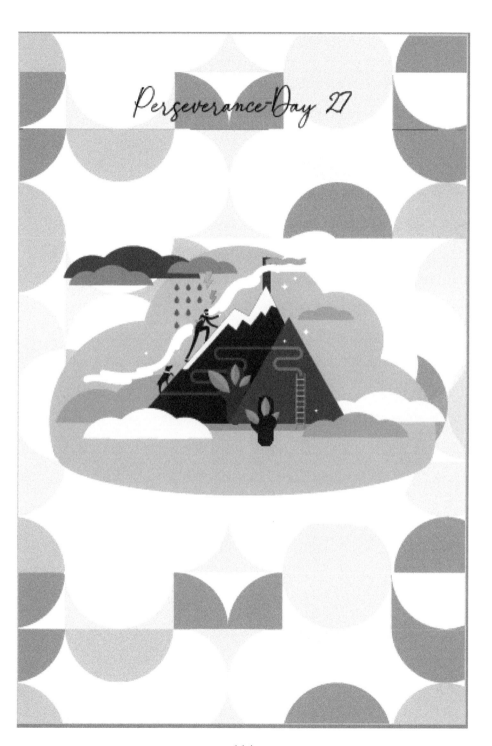

Perseverance – Day 27

News flash….you have successfully made it through every bad day you have ever had. Today will be no different, and you will persevere no matter the circumstances. Life on life's terms is a reality for all of us, and challenges show up without our permission. Applying the principle of perseverance allows us to build confidence in ourselves and our ability to overcome the day-to-day situations that may shake us at the core. Some days you may appear to be a superhero defending the city against villains, and other days you may be holding on by the seat of your pants, counting the minutes until you can go to bed. Regardless of how the day unfolds, we use our strengths and the support of others to persevere. The miracle comes when you lay your head down on the pillow at night in reflection and say, "I made it through another day, and for that I am grateful".

Today's intention routine is very simple. Let's develop a morning narrative of positive perseverance statements to pump ourselves up and become our own cheerleaders. If your pom poms are handy…now is the time to get them out.

Here are a couple of examples:

- I believe in myself and my ability to overcome whatever life throws at me today. I will preserver.

- I will dig deep when challenges arise and draw strength from my inner self.

- I have made it through every bad day I have ever experienced. Today will be the same.

Now take a couple of minutes to write down three of your own positive perseverance statements.

1.) _____

_____

2.) _____

_____

3.) _____

_____

People are watching you, and they will draw strength and hope from your courage to overcome. Now go embrace this day and PERSERVERE…I believe in you!

"I get back up, try again, I realize my perseverance is not only important for myself and my goals, but it's also contagious to those around me. When I stay perseverant, we stay perseverant."

- Daryl Gilmer

Flexibility-Day 28

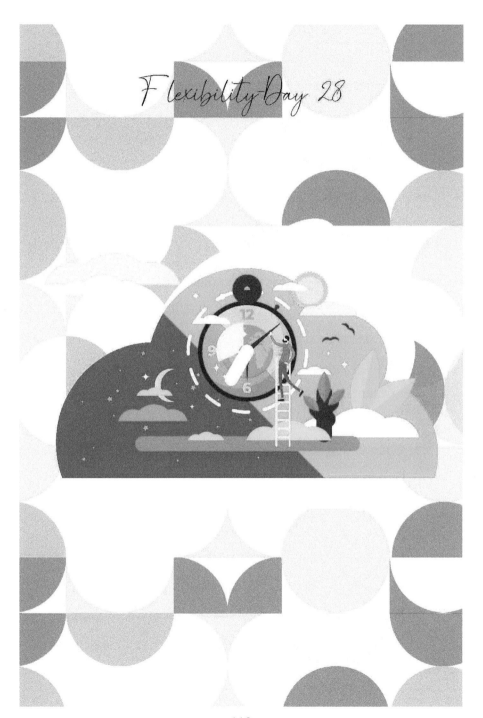

Flexibility – Day 28

Maintaining flexibility with the ebb and flow of life is an essential component of keeping the door open to positivity. A clay pot is malleable and can be reshaped if it remains moist and is stored in the right conditions. Designs, details, a handle, and feet can be added to the pot forever if it isn't sent to the kiln for firing. Once it is sent to the kiln and fired, it becomes ceramic. Consequently, the opportunity for significant change goes away. Paint can be added, but the pot has achieved a very rigid state.

As a result of our experiences, both negative and positive, just like the clay pot, we are slowly molded into the person we are today. It is easy to find beauty in positive experiences and remain willing to grow and change with them. Our experiences with trauma, physical pain, accidents, loss, hurt, break ups, and abuse lead to a negative perspective of life, and make change more of a challenge. Our pain is ours, and we can maintain whatever relationship with it we want. Trauma bonding and avoidant behavior negate us from experiencing the freedom, peace, and serenity we deserve. If we avoid addressing the pain, our hearts will begin to harden, and we will become the ceramic pot. Mehmet Murat Ildan stated, "Life continuously shoots arrows at you; to survive, be flexible and be on the move because rigid and fixed targets are the easiest targets!"

Regardless of the severity of our circumstances, we haven't been sent to the kiln yet, and there is still an opportunity for change. Our willingness to lean into the pain, the courage to preserve through it, and our belief in the healing process will produce positivity. Remaining flexible through the process and open-minded to new ideas sets the table for a life we were created to experience.

Today we will set our intentions to become more flexible and move away from our ridged negative belief system. Take a few minutes to reflect on 2-3 areas of your life you lack flexibility and willingness to change. In the space below, we will briefly identify and explain these areas.

1.)_____

_____

_____

2.)_____

_____

_____

3.)_____

_____

_____

Awareness is the key to change, and pain shared is pain lessened. The simple process of writing these down on paper softens the heart and creates flexibility in our spirits. As a means to speak positivity into our hearts and minds, we will read the positive affirmation narrative below three times out loud.

"I am willing to remain flexible and open to change. I am a malleable piece of clay, who is deserving of a positive mindset and a soft heart. I will achieve freedom from my negative beliefs, because they don't serve me anymore."

Flexibility is the key to positivity, and none of us deserve a life of negativity. Let's live in love today…it's a choice. I believe in you.

"To live in love is life's greatest challenge. It requires more subtlety, flexibility, sensitivity, tolerance, knowledge, and strength than any other human endeavor."

– Leo Buscaglia

I am Me! Day 29

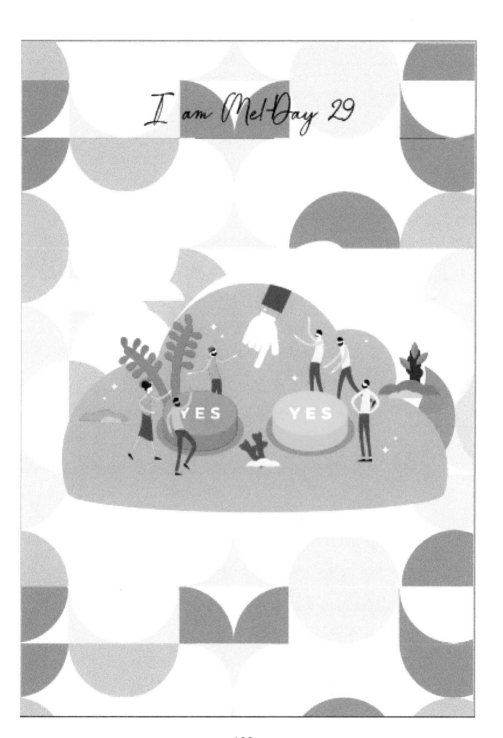

I am Me! – Day 29

Many of us live in a consistent place of "Why me?" Our lives have been filled with a series of events. Some of which have created a tremendous amount of pain and others an abundance of joy. Both have played instrumental roles in the development of our belief system, but our brain's negative bias attaches us tighter to painful events. When bad things happen we ask, "why does this always happen to me?". This comes from an irrational belief that only bad things happen to us and that the rest of the world is free of pain and challenges. The world isn't out to get us, nor are we the only ones feeling pain. If we stay stuck in this negative narrative, we will consequently have challenges accepting any personal responsibility for our path in life and will drown in self-pity. In other cases we ask, "why don't good things happen to me?". The exact nature of this thought commonly comes from a place of insecurity, envy, comparison, and lack of self-worth. These things are developed in childhood and validated by the people around us, and our own internal dialogue as we mature.

Moving from a place of "why me", towards "I am me", is a foundational piece of the puzzle on the road to producing positivity. We empower ourselves to take control of our destiny with an, "I am me!" mentality. This helps us move away from comparison and towards creativity. The world provides us with a huge canvas and the opportunity to create our own masterpieces. We are autonomous in choosing the colors, patterns, designs, and details. Holding onto our false beliefs or skewed perceptions may inhibit us from even picking up the paintbrush. Jackson Pollock said, "Every good painter paints what he is." Letting go of what we think we are, opens the door to creating who we want to be.

Today we will set out with the intention of creating our own masterpiece. We will start by shifting to a more positive perspective. Below we will list five positive things we currently have in our lives that we intend to keep as part of the masterpiece. These can be family, friends, career, love, God, spirituality, hobbies, etc. We will also list five new things we would like to add to our masterpiece. Examples of these could be self-care, exercise, career change, reunification with family, relationships, travel, healing trauma, boundaries, children, etc.

Currently parts of Masterpiece	Future parts of Masterpiece

We will now use the blank space provided to bring our masterpieces together in a work of art. None of us are Van Gogh or Picasso, so stick figures will work. If the thought of any sort of art makes you cringe, using words with different colors and sizes will work. Our intention is to define what we want our life to look like, and a vision we can work towards. Dig deep for your inner kindergartener and begin. Crayons are acceptable, throwing a temper tantrum isn't.

Our life is in a constant state of change, and things happen with and without our permission. Our path toward positivity is dependent on taking ownership of what we have control over and letting the rest go. We lead with "I am me" and quit asking why not me. Remember, we are holding our own paintbrush. Let's do this....I believe in you.

"When one door of happiness closes, another opens; but often we look so long at the closed door that we do not see the one which has been opened for us."

- Helen Keller

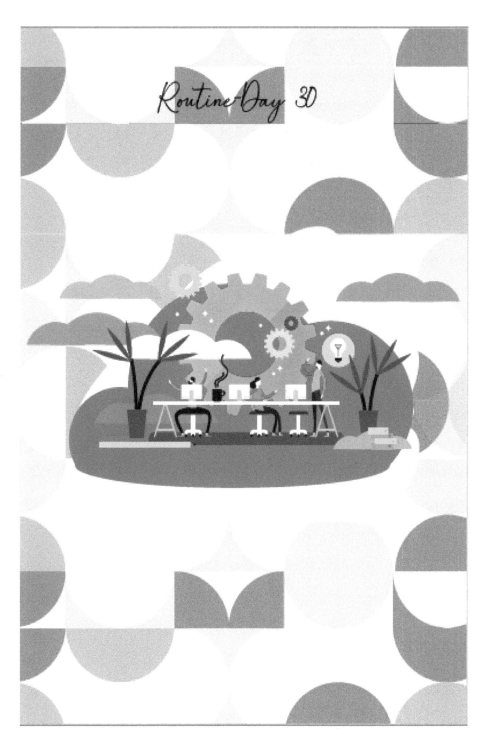

Routine Day 3D

Routine – Day 30

A routine is an essential component of a life filed with positivity and peace. Throughout this book, several seeds have been planted in our lives. In order for these seeds to grow and establish roots, they must be watered on a scheduled routine. We water these seeds by actively engaging in activities on a regular basis. We maintain change through commitment, action, and consistency. If we have found a more positive perspective of ourselves through affirmation work, we must continue this work to experience the results. A gratitude list for seven days will only create an attitude of gratitude temporarily. The benefits of mindful meditation will only exist when we are actively engaged in our practice. The self-enrichment process we have started will only manifest if we continue to seek out knowledge through research, reading new material, intellectual conversations, and enriching activities. We will only maintain our overall health, nutritional health, and physical fitness if we continue to make diet and exercise important and maintain a routine. Aristotle said, "We are what we repeatedly do." Repetition creates a new direction and a new version of us.

Our intention for today is to establish a routine we can commit to and complete daily. We must set realistic expectations of ourselves, or we will fail. This routine can be changed in the future if our circumstances or abilities change. This is a commitment to ourselves to continue to practice courage, perseverance, and willingness long into the future. Use the space below to create a daily routine you can commit to for at least 30 days, and then reevaluate your progress. This can be a morning routine, a routine you do throughout the day, or an evening routine. When you do it, isn't as important as making sure you get it done.

Example: I wake up every morning and actively engage in a morning routine. I start with a brief meditation. Then I journal, write a gratitude list, and sit in self-reflection. I complete all of these every day before I enter the world. When I am done, I am spiritually centered and more equipped for life on life's terms.

———————————————————

———————————————————

———————————————————

———————————————————

———————————————————

———————————————————

———————————————————

This new routine is a recipe for a new positive you. I believe in you, and I am excited about the positive changes you will see in your life.

"Schedules are meant to help, not hinder. Create them with your lifestyle in mind."

– Chrissy Halton

Action Day 3

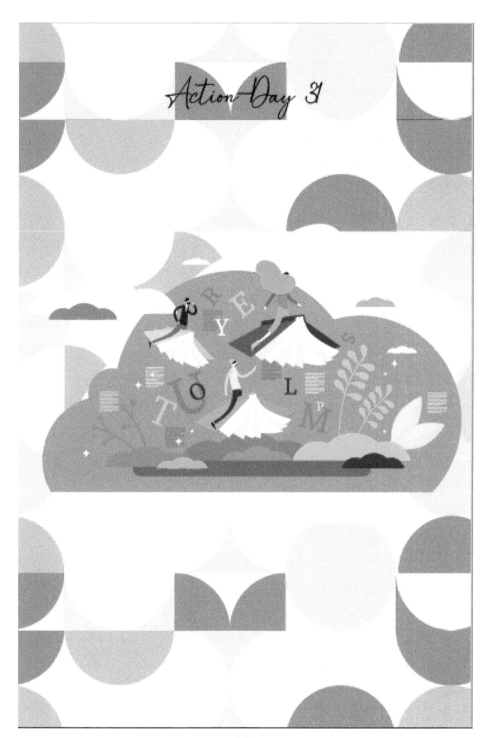

Action – Day 31

Each day for the last 30 days, we have set our intentions to create change in our lives. The simple act of setting intentions is an action, but only the beginning. The hope is after we set our intentions, it is followed up by living with purpose throughout the day. Intentions only generate direction, not the end results. In order to produce positive results in our lives, we must get into "positive action". At this point in the journey we have established various tasks and skills to use in varying ways. Some of these may have created significant change in our lives, and we may have picked up momentum. In order to maintain the changes, we must continue to engage in the activities that created them. Nothing will happen by osmosis, or if we merely intend for change to happen. Positive action renders positive results. Catherine Pulsifer stated, "We all find ourselves in situations that at times seem hopeless. And, we all have the choice to do nothing or take action." Let's choose action…it beats the alternative.

Today we set our intentions to continue this process of daily self-love and action well into the future. There is a space below to identify the three most impactful tools you have added to your tool belt, and how you will apply them regularly.

For example, "I have been intentional with my positive self-talk every day and it has improved my perspective of myself. I will continue to do this daily even when I feel good about myself." Lets do this...I believe in you!

1.)_____

_____

_____

_____

2.)_____

_____

_____

_____

3.)_____

_____

_____

_____

"A man is the sum of his actions, of what he has done, of what he can do. Nothing else."

– Gandhi

Conclusion

We made it! A 31-day commitment to living with intention, practicing self-love, and producing positivity. The hope is we feel accomplished and ready to continue down the path of positivity. The journey doesn't stop here. It has only begun. We now have a responsibility to ourselves to maintain our aim in the direction we desire our life to go. Anthony Covington wrote, "Accomplishment changes the hearts and minds of those encouraged by it," and "It can motivate right thinking because it brings about what we think about. We are always accomplishing our aim. What are you aiming for?"

The intention of this book was to refocus our aim and live with intention. Practice doesn't make us perfect, but it provides the opportunity for growth. Our negative beliefs, thinking, and behaviors have been identified through this process, and we have given birth to a new perspective. We have been provided with an assortment of simple tasks we can utilize to maintain the change and avoid relapsing into the old version of ourselves. Not every suggested task throughout the 31 day process is for everyone. We eat the chicken and spit out the bones. For our vegan and vegetarian friends, just eat the cherries and spit out the seeds. We take what we have benefited from, add it to our tool belt, and leave the rest behind.

The journey to positivity can be rough and painful. There will be days when giving up seems like our only option. It is an option, but it isn't a solution. Spending a day on the couch with a bag of potato chips is okay occasionally, but this is only a temporary fix to a continuous problem. We are strong, powerful, courageous, and intelligent people who have been given the opportunity to impact our lives and those around us in magical ways. We no longer need to live a life of negativity. It is time we lean into the pain and discomfort of change and embrace the beauty that comes from it. I will leave you with the metaphor of the buffalo and cow in hopes to inspire you on your journey to positivity.

When we think of buffaloes and cows, we identify a lot of similarities. They both graze in open pastures for food, have hooves, and horns, remain with the herd, and are herbivores. One interesting fact separating them is how they respond in the presence of a storm. When a storm arrives, cows inherently begin to run away from the storm. One may think this is a great way to avoid getting pounded by heavy rains, turbulent winds, and heavy snow. Unfortunately, after a period of time the cows begin to get tired, and the storm continues to come. Consequently, the cow becomes overwhelmed by the power of the storm and has nowhere to go. This is very similar to what we as humans experience when we avoid painful or stressful situations. We turn and run in the face of adversity to minimize the severity of the pain. Just like the cow, we can only run from the pain for so long before it begins to overwhelm us.

Buffalo on the other hand, run fearlessly straight into the center of the storm as soon as they feel it is coming. Many of us may think this is crazy and reckless, but it is actually very wise and courageous. The buffalo will initially get pounded by the force of the storm but will come out the other side faster. On the other side of every storm is typically bright and peaceful skies. The period the buffalo experiences pain is much less than that of the cow. Running into the storms of life isn't always comfortable, but it beats getting pounded repeatedly. We need to live our lives more like buffalo and lean into discomfort. Running away only prolongs the pain. Facing it produces a positive path to peace, freedom, and growth. Ultimately leading to emotional strength and maturity. Be the buffalo, not the cow!

True change occurs when the belief in ourselves and our worthiness of a positive life provokes the desire in our spirit to maintain our path of positivity.

I believe in you, and you are worthy of a beautiful and positive life. The journey isn't over. It has only begun. Let's do this…it beats the alternative.

Notes